How To

Lose Weight

And

Stay Fit

Diana De Rose

ACKNOWLEDGEMENTS

I would like to thank my parents for teaching me the importance of a healthy body. My dad for encouraging me to stay fit and my mom for her constant nagging to eat healthy. To my brother, hope you follow at least two chapters of this book.

To my husband Jose for being a constant support he has always been and for bearing with all my experiments about losing weight.

To all my friends and relatives, who have taught me in some way or the other, the art of eating healthy and staying fit.

This section will be incomplete without thanking Amazon and CreateSpace for providing such a wonderful medium to self-publish this book.

Lastly to all my readers - Stay healthy, stay fit!!!

And to everyone else not mentioned here but did play a role in contributing to this book - Thank you.

Diana De Rose

Author's Note

First of all I will begin by saying that I am not a doctor nor a physicist or dietician or any other fitness trainer. I am just a person who likes to stay fit. Weight loss has intimidated more than 50% of world population. We all at some point of our life have tried to lose weight, sometimes we are successful, sometimes we are not and sometimes it is much more than that.

People often focus on the wrong goal. They worry about losing weight but forget about staying fit in the process. During the early half of my life I have made many such mistakes too. Some of these mistakes affected me physically and some emotionally. We as humans have a tendency to follow others and we often end up measuring ourselves based on other people's metrics. "All size doesn't fit all", these wonderful words are quite true in this aspect.

This book is my attempt to help people realize how easy it is to lose weight but at the same time how important it is to stay healthy. Feeling good about yourself and how you look is as important as anything else that you are about to do. Focusing on the bigger picture is the key to achieving this goal. Eating right is an art, come let us explore it.

How this book works:

The chapters in this book are divided into three sections:

1. Fundamentals: This section builds the foundation of the art. I do not call it diet because I feel this is a negative word and is very ambiguous. This section helps you understand your body in a better way as well as the chemistry of the foods that we consume. There are some astonishing numbers here, feel free to skip them if it intimidates you.

2. Action: This section is all about getting into action. It helps in providing you with a plan that works best for your body and schedule. I have shared few important Tips in this section that you should consider following. There are plenty of practical examples as well.

3. Maintain: Like everything else, body also requires maintenance. Human body is like a machine which works well when all of its organs function harmoniously. Doing wrong things can cause these organs to behave abnormally. It is easy to achieve success but very difficult to maintain it. This section helps you maintain what you achieved from the above two sections.

Who should not use this book:

Finally, word of caution for those who should not be using this book. All are welcome to read it but not everyone may be able to apply the principles mentioned here. Here is why I think you should not read this:

1. If you have long term illness or are pregnant.

2. People who are obese and think reading this book is the silver bullet to losing weight in a month.

3. People who are in a quest to achieve size zero figure.

4. Those who consider losing weight as a onetime activity.

Lastly, at the end of the book, there is a section dedicated to topics that I couldn't cover. I have this section in all my books. I would love to hear back from all my readers if you have any suggestions and or ideas that you think needs to be shared with others.

My email address is present at the end of the book. You are all welcome to write to me, send your feedback and any other suggestions that you have and I will include it in the book in a future version.

Thank you.

Diana De Rose

Jan 2014

CONTENTS

1

1. COMMITMENT AND DETERMINATION

Like any of your other goals, losing weight also requires commitment and determination to a very large extent. Sometimes much more than what you require for your regular goal. It tests your patience, temptations, your inhibitions, weaknesses and everything else. Contrary to other goals, losing weight requires quite a lot of hard work and patience, if not it can lead to negative effects.

Losing weight is not an overnight activity. You cannot drink a magic potion and expect to become slim the next day. Print that last phrase and stick it on the wall of your bedroom or read it out loud at least ten times, so that it sticks to your memory forever. Weight loss requires time; it requires lots and lots of patience.

But do not worry. Together through this book, we will learn the five essential steps to a simple and healthy weight loss program that is custom made for each one of us. And yes, you do not have to follow what others do or say, not even what I say. You make your own regimen. The key to success is in doing things that you like. My principle is to make you mix your flour and bake the cake. Only then you will be able to eat it, no matter how bad it is. That being said, this is the last time we will be talking about cake in this book. Let's get to some work now.

First and foremost, here are the five steps to feeling good. Yes, I do not call it weight loss; I call it the feel good regimen because at the end of this, all I want you to achieve is feeling good about yourself. Detail explanation on each of these goals is provided in the rest of the book.

1. Goal:

One of the first things to do is to find out what your actual goal is. I know losing weight is your end goal but it's not as simple as it appears. We need to get into the specifics. What is your current weight, how much do you want to reduce, do you want to build muscles? Are you doing it to avoid other medical condition such as reducing sugar and cholesterol levels?

What is the end result you are expecting from your activity? Most of us start off on our weight loss program without knowing what we are trying to achieve. Getting your goal clear is the first step to achieving it. Spend a day or two, perhaps even a week to establish that. Give proper thought and write down your goals.

2. Plan:

The next step is to come up with an ideal plan. Planning is one of the most important parts of your weight loss regimen. Take a look at your life, your daily schedule, your body. Some people make very aggressive schedule like going on a no carb diet, paleo diet, liquid diet, working out for more than eight hours, cabbage soup diet and so on without even investigating if that is the right thing for you.

Trust me, these do not work. You cannot eat less if you are doing high physical activity every day. Take it slow. An ideal plan doesn't develop in a day. It involves lots of experimenting and lots of trial and error. Focus on increasing your metabolism rather than decreasing your food intake.

3. Prepare

Next step is to prepare a regimen that best works for you. Keep in mind that this is not the only thing you will be doing in the next few months. You need to take an account of your daily work, personal healthcare, other commitments and most important the fact that you do not get bored or stop following your own regimen.

One of the key things to keep in mind is to take one step at a time. Start by small things like reducing sugar in your coffee or tea from 2tsp to 1 or 1/2tsp. Then slowly increase it to reducing the sugar altogether, getting rid of fats, refined food from your diet and so on. Make a plan that is doable.

4. Follow

Follow the plan religiously. Let nothing come on the way to your healthy regimen. Weather, friends, party, vacation, weekend, work, all these are just excuses to being lazy. Think of it as something that you have to do. If you cannot give up eating, drinking and shower for anything else, you should not give up this regimen too.

If you have prior commitments, account for it when you make your regimen. That's where proper planning comes into picture. Do not take anything lightly.

5. Maintain

This is the last and the most important step. Most of us achieve what we want within a few months but then we lose focus, we become lazy and give up our good habits. We go back to how we were before and ruin all our past efforts. You can be less aggressive once you achieve your goal but you should not stop following good habits. Good practices should continue forever.

Now that we know the five steps to achieving our goal, let's get into some action in the next chapters.

2

2. FOCUS ON WHAT YOU EAT

Do you eat to live or live to eat? We might have heard this sentence many times earlier but probably never paid much attention to its importance. Answering the question to the above sentence can help you know where you stand.

Few years ago a colleague asked me how am I able to limit my diet. I replied that I don't fancy food the same way as she does. I consider it as something we need to consume to stay alive, consider it as a chore that we must do every day just like brushing teeth, taking shower and other similar activities. One does not brush ten times a day just because toothpaste tastes good or one doesn't take a shower four times a day just because they have a nice bathroom. Same way just because the food tastes so good, it doesn't mean one has to eat a lot.

By now you are already aware that food plays an important role on your weight. Just paying close attention on what you eat can do the trick in most cases. The key is to eat healthy, eat enough. Eating more or less that what you require can cause adverse effects. Eat larger portions earlier in the day and reduce it as the day goes by.

Some things to avoid:

1. Binge eating - eating just because there is lot of food left.

2. Eating too late in the night in large quantities.

3. Eating refined foods - like canned, frozen meals, ready to eat food.

4. Low fat foods

5. Stay away from anything that is fried

6. Loading up on sugar - candies, juice, and soda.

7. Living on soda

Some things to adapt:

1. Eat more fruits

2. Eat more vegetables - Add lots of raw vegetables to your diet if possible like cucumber, spinach, carrot, and avocado.

3. Eat more fish

4. Use good fats like olive oil

5. Snacks on nuts and dried fruits - although make sure there aren't too much sugar on them.

6. Drink lots of water - more on this in a later chapter.

7. Eat whole grains as opposed to white bread or pasta or rice.

Summary to natural weight loss food

1. Eat more protein, fiber, and healthy fats. This means more lean meats, vegetables, fruits and nuts.

2. Eat less junk, refined and sugary foods. These are the worst enemies of your body, and they are often the cause of many other chronic diseases like diabetes, hypertension, etc.

3. Drink more water, at least two liters a day is a bare minimum. Less than that and your body will not be able to burn fat most efficiently.

3

3. THE LOW FAT CALORIE DIET

The other day I read an interesting book on the misconception people have about the low fat calorie food. A lot of people in the US are obese. For a country that spends the highest amount of money on health care we are not necessarily healthy. A large population of US has cancer, heart diseases and other cardiovascular diseases. We also have one of the highest rates of child diabetes.

And to fight all that about two decades ago the low fat food was introduced in the market. Today if you visit a grocery store you will be able to find low fat versions of pretty much everything - low fat candy, low fat coffee, low fat cream, low fat cereal, low fat meat etc. (I am glad there isn't any low fat vegetable out there yet)

The reason we find so many low fat products is because it is successful among people. People blindly follow it without knowing the real meaning about it. They think that eating low fat is healthy but they fail to realize that if low fat products were introduced two decades ago then why are there still so many cases of obesity? Why are people falling ill? Why were people in olden days not obese or had a higher life span even after eating food rich in fats? The answer is very simple. It is not the fat that is unhealthy; it is the sugar that we eat which is bad.

The other day I read an article which says that according to the quality inspection norms if a product has less than 0.2 gm of an ingredient in the sample size then you can market it as 0gm.

So for example if your peanut butter contains 0.2 gm of sugar in 2tsp (30gm) sample, the company is allowed to market it as 0% sugar or sugar free. People get mislead by the 0 sugar and buy the product. And when you consume the same peanut butter, I am sure no one uses just 2tsp in their spread. Let's assume you used 5tsp or probably more feeling happy that you can consume more now guilt free but what you are really consuming is about 1-2gm of sugar when you actually thought you were consuming none.

For those who think that 1-2gm is probably not going to cost you much in terms of health, you may be right if you really watch your sugar intake but when you learn about the various ways through which sugar gets into your body, you will start to worry.

A lot of people consume skim milk instead of whole milk thinking low fat is good. Pasteurized skim milk isn't a great choice either. Because the fat is removed and much of the nutrition is destroyed during pasteurization, there is not much left except for milk and sugar.

Egg whites: There is a popular misconception among people that they are eating healthy by having egg whites. What most of us don't know is that all the nutrition of the egg resides in the yolk. It has protein and various other vitamins which gets lost when you throw away the yellow and eat just white. Instead have eggs in moderation. Having one or two egg a day will not cause any problem.

Fats are essential for our body. Having low fat food actually causes our body to produce more insulin which causes the body to crave for more sugar. Low fat food deprives the body of essential nutrients which in turn causes more fatigue and reduces the metabolism.

The best way to eat healthy is to eat what has been around for hundreds of years, what our ancestors used to eat who obviously were healthier. Stick to whole grains, fruits and veggies and do not consider meat as bad, meat is important too.

The key is not to over eat one particular thing. Anything in excess is bad. Reduce the amount of processed food in your diet and incorporate more of raw or home cooked meals in your diet. I am sure with these few changes life would really be amazing.

4

4. REMOVE SUGAR

There is a reason food expert and nutritionists ask you to stay low on sugar. Of all the things that you eat every day, sugar is probably the most dangerous one and also the one that you should pay the most attention to. Other than the obvious fact that excess of sugar causes tooth decay, it also makes you gain weight by adding bad fat. Sugar comes in various forms, not just the table sugar that you see.

Sugars are a type of carbohydrates. It is a complex food containing glucose, fructose and sucrose. It is not easily breakable by the body hence high intake of sugar causes our body to store it as fat. What happens next? When your pancreas detects a rush of sugar, it releases a hormone called insulin to deal with all of that excess sugar. Insulin helps store all of this glucose in the liver and muscles but often our body struggles to get that balance right. This results in too much insulin being released, which ultimately results in our blood sugar dropping below normal levels. This causes a sugar rush and we end up craving more sugar and the cycle goes on.

Let us look at a list of items that goes into the body as sugar:

1. Bread

2. Rice, pasta, noodles

3. Juice - raw as well as bottled/canned

4. Beverages

5. Nutrition bars

6. Alcohol

7. Cookies and candies

How to identify sugar in your food:

Read the label in everything that you buy. Look for the words ending with -ose Sucrose, Maltose, Dextrose, Fructose, Glucose, Galactose, Lactose, High fructose corn syrup, Glucose solids. Just because it doesn't end in -ose, however, doesn't mean it isn't sugar. There are plenty of other names as well that may or may not sound like sugar.

Regardless of how they sound, the following are all sugar:

Cane juice, Dehydrated cane juice, Cane juice solids, Cane juice crystals, Dextrin, Maltodextrin, Dextran, Barley malt, Beet sugar, Corn syrup, Corn syrup solids, Caramel, Buttered syrup, Carob syrup, Brown sugar, Date sugar, Malt syrup, Diastase, Diatastic malt, Fruit juice, Fruit juice concentrate, Dehydrated fruit juice, Fruit juice crystals, Golden syrup, Turbinado, Sorghum syrup, Refiner's syrup, Ethyl maltol, Maple syrup, Yellow sugar

It doesn't take a lot of time to identify sugar in your diet. Just taking a look at the ingredient list of all items you buy can do the trick.

5

5. ADD VARIETY

Add variety to your food. Eating healthy foods can be boring. As much as we would love to eat fried potatoes, chicken nuggets and hamburgers every day, we all know that is not the right way to go. The only way to motivate yourself into eating healthy is by adding variety to your diet.

Just because you like one particular vegetable doesn't mean that you have to eat that every day. Likewise if you like having tuna salad for lunch doesn't mean you need to have tuna salad for lunch for the rest of your life. We all like some food and do not like certain foods but that shouldn't keep us from trying different things. The key to not getting bored of following your routine is by adding variety to your diet.

Make pasta one day, baked fish another day, try a mushroom soup the week after. Google healthy recipes and you will find tons of healthy recipes to try. Eating healthy doesn't necessarily mean eating boring food consisting of salad and fruits every day.

Also add a variety of fruits to your diet. I never used to take fruits until I was in my mid-twenties. But once I realized the benefits of fruit, I started incorporating it in my everyday diet sometimes more than one fruit every day.

Each week I buy a different fruit especially the ones that in season. Try local farm produced vegetables. There are lots of vegetables that are native to the place you live. There are certain vegetables and fruits that you won't find if you travel outside of your city or country. Try to relish them.

Tip: Try eating fruits that are in season as opposed to fruits that you like but are not in season. The simple reason being fruits that are not in season but available in the market is probably been grown artificially to make it available year round. That's the last thing you want to put in your stomach, harmful chemicals. Also buying seasonal fruits will be easy on your wallet.

Same goes with vegetables too. Buy seasonal vegetables; try to incorporate a few raw veggies if possible in the form of salads, guacamole, chutneys, dips etc.

6

6. ADD COLOR

Continuing with what we learnt in the last chapter about adding variety brings us to another important concept of adding color to your diet. Now this may seem misleading if you read it literally. But by adding color I am not implying to use artificial food coloring to your diet instead I am asking you to add fruits and vegetables of different color.

When you grab your lunch make sure your plate has at least four colors - red, green, brown, white. Well not really in that order, what I really want you to do is include fruits(red), vegetables(green), grains(brown) and meat(white). You can play with as many colors as you like as long as you get the point.

Now I know fruits can contain a lot of fructose (and thus a lot of sugar). That being said, I believe that consumption of fruit can be beneficial. When you consume fruit, you are not only consuming fructose (in its natural state), but also consuming fiber and lots of vitamins and minerals. Yes, fruit can have an effect on your blood sugar, it is sugar after all. But generally fruit will cause less of a blood sugar spike compared to table sugar or high fructose corn syrup.

In addition to that, fiber also plays an important part of a balanced diet (ask your bowels), and fruit can contain a lot of it.

Tip: Try to eat fruits with skin on them as they are a good source of fiber. Also wash fruits thoroughly before eating.

Now we all know fruits are healthy but what about fruit juices? Lot of people drink fruit juice every day and feel very happy about it. Well when it comes to weight loss and reducing sugar content, fruit juices are an absolute no.

Here is why: When you consume fruit juices like orange juice, apple juice, or cranberry juice, the juice is squeezed, giving you all of the juice but very little of the fiber or nutrients that get left behind in the process. And most juices are loaded with sugar to give the sweet flavor.

Some stats from various sources:

Orange juice - 21g of sugar

Apple juice - 28g of sugar

Cranberry juice - 37g of sugar

Grape juice - 38g of sugar

Coca-Cola - 40g of sugar.

If you are going to eat fruit, get it in fruit form, not juice form. If you are going to drink juice, squeeze it yourself, and even then consume it in small quantities.

Tip: When you make your own juice, do not add sugar.

Let's talk a little bit about vegetables before we end this chapter. Most vegetables are green in color and some of the best one's are the leafy ones likes spinach, kale, cabbage, broccoli, green beans. That being said, it doesn't mean other colored vegetables like red and yellow pepper, eggplant, pumpkin, cauliflower, carrots and beets are not good. Each of these other colored vegetables has their own bonus nutrients and it's best to include them in your diet regularly.

Tip: Most vegetables taste good if you steam/boil and sauté those with olive oil and sprinkle little bit of salt and pepper.

What about grains? I cannot finish this chapter without talking about grains. For some people grains are an important part of their daily diet and they cannot replace it with anything. Well good news, you don't have to cut grains out of your diet, instead substitute it with healthy alternatives. For example if you like white rice, substitute it with brown rice, if you like bread then eat whole grain wheat bread instead of white bread, same goes for pasta too. Also try to experiment with grains such as couscous, millet, and quinoa. These grains though not widely used but are considered very healthy.

.

7

7. EAT HEALTHY FATS

Fats are all not bad. Fats are categorized into two categories - good fats and bad fats. The good fats are essential fats that are required by our body to stay healthy. Before getting into details of good fat and bad fat, let me first explain why fat is essential for us.

Fats are like reserved food stored by our body as a failback mechanism for the rainy day. In the event of sickness or energy loss, your body uses these fats to get going. However due to the popular misconception among people that all fats are bad, it is easy for people to lack these wonderful reserved fats. In fact 20-30% of your daily calories must come from fats. So let's get into some details.

1. Good fat: (or as technical people call them Monosaturated fats)

These fats increase the good cholesterol (HDL) level in your body and decrease the bad cholesterol (LDL). I won't go into the details for HDL and LDL here because it will get too technical and I want to keep this book as simple as possible. However, if you are interested in knowing more about these, there is an elaborate article in Wikipedia about it.

So what do these fats do? Well, they protect the body against the buildup of substance that clogs your arteries. They also boost brain function and help strengthen the immune system and improve mood swings as well as keep skin and eyes healthy.

How to get them: Healthy oils such as olive oil, canola oil, healthy nuts such as almonds, cashews, peanuts, peanut butter, flaxseed, walnuts, sesame seeds, and vegetables such as avocados and seafood such as in fish like salmon, mackerel and in tofu. Although these fats are healthy, one must remember not to over consume these foods. Excess of anything is bad and so is the case with good fats.

2. Bad fat: (also known as Saturated fats)

Needless to say these fats increases your cholesterol levels and raise the risk of heart diseases and various other illness.

How do you get them: It is easier than you think in most cases. These fats are widely found in the form of meats such as pork, beef and even chicken. Yes, you heard it right white meat is not good either. Other sources are butter, cream, milk, coconut oil etc. Well, that doesn't mean that you should become vegetarian.

A good point to start is by removing all kinds of visible fat from what you eat like for example removing the skin of the chicken, prefer grilled meat as opposed to fried meat, limit red meat to one or two times a week, remove butter and cream from daily cooking and use it only for special occasions.

With these small changes in your lifestyle you can easily reduce if not replace the bad fats in your body. One good habit to adapt is to become a pescetarian at least on weekdays. I try to follow that. I eat seafood all throughout the week and eat meat on weekends if necessary. That way I don't give up meat and also get my good fats into the body.

8

8. WHEN QUICK BITE BECOMES LARGER

Ever been in a situation where you wanted to grab something quick and you ended up having an elaborate meal? Not just that, sometimes when we are not very hungry and grab a small bite hoping to calm the hunger down, only to regret it later as the small bite triggered your appetite and made you want even more.

Believe it or not, controlling what you eat is one of the most difficult activities most people face. Almost everyone has some kind of addiction. Addictions come in different ways, it could be chocolate, it could be soda, and it could be chips, coffee or anything else.

That doesn't mean that having control on one's diet is an impossible thing. I have known many people who have very good control over food. One of the easiest ways to practice self-control is to pick one item every week or month and try to not eat them. Pick something that you like and are likely to be in a situation where you might be tempted to eat.

Where people go wrong:

Many people try to give up lot of things at the same time. For example they cut carbs, sugar, soda, desserts all at the same time. When that happens, you end up losing your control, temptation kicks in and you start eating everything back again. The point is to try to remove items one at a time.

The solution to healthy living is not by giving away what you like but to eat small portions of it. The main test is to make sure that you do not eat larger portions of the same food all the time. There are also studies that show that eating small six meals is better than having three large meals.

Although I haven't tried that but I do believe in eating large portions earlier in the day and reduce it towards the night. However not all size fits one when it comes to food. Every person's body behaves in a different way to different food items, the only way you can be sure of your body is to try to different things and see what works best for you.

9

9. BUY A WEIGHING SCALE

There are some things that you should always have in your home one of which is a weighing scale. Investing in a nice weighing scale is one of the best things I have ever done. Many people underestimate the importance of weighing scale. It not only helps you know your weight but also acts as a constant reminder to keep the weight in check.

The best place to keep your weighing machine is in your bathroom. Most people go to the bathroom first thing in the morning. Well here is what you can do. Every morning after you wake up, go to the bathroom, clear your stomach and weigh yourself before you shower. Body weight increases and decreases throughout the day based on what we eat and what we do. Hence measuring the weight at different times of the day can give you a wrong indication of your weight. In the morning when you wake up, all your food from previous day is well digested hence the weight you measure in the morning is your true weight.

Have a weighing machine and start measuring your weight everyday first thing in the morning. Start by weighing yourself at various times in the day to monitor how your body weight increases throughout the day. Weighing yourself daily motivates you to maintain your weight. It also helps you identify what foods causes your weight to increase drastically and what physical activity helps you reduce weight. Weighing yourself is a good addiction but try to not to get obsessed with it.

In the initial phase weigh at least four times a day and later reduce it to one or two times a day, once in the morning and once before bed. After all, the last thing you want is to be called an obsessive compulsive weight conscious person.

Weighing machine is also a good gift for a friend but make sure you do not offend them by giving it to them. When my parents visited me few years back, they got addicted to my weighing scale so much that at the end of their three month trip they had each lost 5-10 pounds. And they insisted me on gifting them a weighing scale as a going away gift. That is one gift they still treasure.

10

10. CREATE YOUR OWN PHYSICAL

REGIMEN

This is the fun part, creating your own daily regime. Isn't it nice, you do not have to pay anyone to do this for you. After all who knows your body better than you? This is probably one of the most difficult steps of your weight loss activity for obvious reasons of course.

Well first and foremost you should be keep in mind that this is a developing regime and you will have to include or reduce things in this regimen as you move ahead. One size doesn't fit all; same way what works for you may not work for your brother or friend. So you should be very careful. Let's get started.

1. **Plan your breakfast:** Let's start with breakfast since this is the first and most important meal of the day. I always make it a point to include protein, carbs, fat and vitamins in my breakfast. Now that may sound intimidating but it isn't.

For example whole wheat toast, egg, some seasonal fruits, having just these three things can help you get all of the above. Avoid using butter in your toast, use feta cheese instead if you must have cheese. Avoid fruit juices and have real fruits instead. At no cost use white bread, always use wheat and yes you can eat the whole egg. Some people just have egg white but that isn't necessary unless you are eating more than three eggs a day. If you are making an omelet use olive oil and add tomatoes and bell peppers too if possible. Stay away from cheese and sausage or bacon, if you must have it; consume it on only one day preferably Sunday.

2. **Physical activity:** Make sure no matter what happens you include 30 minutes of physical activity in your day excluding your usual walk at work, at home and other chores that you do. You can use these 30 minutes in the gym, walking, running, playing, swimming or any other way. Just make sure to spend just 30 minutes each day. You do not have to wake up at 5am in the morning to do this. You can do it at any time as long as you do it.

3. **Eat well:** At no cost skip your meals. You will be doing yourself a huge favor by following this simple rule. Eat three proper meals a day. Important point here is portion control. One easy way to do that is by eating in a bowl as opposed to plate. Chew your food well. Read that sentence again, and say it out loud. Chew your food well.

Be aware of what you are eating and relish every moment of it. This is very important. And here is why. Hunger is a signal sent to the brain from your stomach. If you eat too fast, your brain doesn't get the signal of being satiated; hence you keep eating until you are bloated. When you chew and eat slowly, you are sending signals to your brain simultaneously as you eat; hence the brain gets the signal faster.

Try it out yourself and you will see the difference. Eating slowing and chewing well also aids in digestion which improves your overall health. And no, we are not cheating the brain here; we are only helping it get the message faster.

4. **Snack:** Snacks are important part of our life and we should not skip them either. Although if you eat well, you shouldn't be feeling the need of a snack but sometimes we do feel the need and here is what you can do. Whenever you are hungry between meals, try to drink water as much as you can. In fact drink water even when you are not hungry. If you are still hungry, get a non-sugar loaded beverage like tea or coffee. If you really want to munch on something then munch on dried nuts, popcorn, fruits or good oat based organic energy bar or a whole wheat peanut butter sandwich with no jelly. Whatever you do, try not to resort to cookies or chips or soda at any cost. These will kill your regimen that very moment.

5. **Sleep:** Sleep is very important for your mental and emotional health. We all know that human body requires eight hours of sleep, so I won't stress the importance of this anymore. I added this point here to make sure you account for it in your daily regime.

6. **Misc.:** There are other miscellaneous activities that you need to address like using the stairs whenever possible, walking instead of taking the car if your destination is within one mile. Get up from your desk as frequently as possible, for example instead of calling your colleague on messenger or phone walk to their place. Do not eat at your desk. Walk to the cafeteria or the nearby park during lunch break. Basically do not sit at one place for more than an hour. Keep moving whenever possible.

Incorporating the above activities will help you build a good regimen. No matter how you do it, make sure it is pleasurable. Own this regimen. Like in project management terms, you are the product owner here. You need to make sure you understand the requirements and the work gets done.

11

11. Do not focus on eating less, focus on improving your metabolism

We have almost finished reading 10 chapters so far and I am sure you would have guessed by now that losing weight is not about eating less. It is about eating right and of course improving your metabolism. Let's first define metabolism for the benefit of those who aren't very familiar with it. In simple terms it is the process by which the body breaks down the food and produces energy which is then transported to various cells and consumed by the body. The faster your metabolism, the more all your food will be used by your body for energy, more calories will be burnt and more pounds will be lost. On the other hand slower metabolism will lead to lesser breakdown of food and more accumulation of fat.

Every person has different levels of metabolism and metabolism does change with age. Starting at about age 25, the average person's metabolism declines between 5% and 10% per decade. That's not good news because we aren't getting any younger however improving metabolism is not rocket science either. Let's first see what causes metabolism to slow down.

Metabolism slows down when body has less energy. Metabolism as we know is the process of breaking food into energy, which means if your body is running low on energy, it will try to conserve the energy by slowing down the metabolism. Some of the examples of body having low energy are due to lack of sleep, skipping meals, living on junk food or low fat diet.

How can you increase your metabolism? That is very important question with a very simple solution. Just eat right and get plenty of sleep. Some foods that specifically improve metabolism are fish which contains omega 3 fatty acids; caffeine also helps in boasting metabolism and its best if taken in the morning. Other examples are green tea and hot peppers. I wouldn't advocate on indulging on the latter three. But no matter what route you pick remember the simple rule - do not over do.

Other activities that improve metabolism are drinking plenty of water. Luke warm is best and of course lots of physical activity. What are you waiting for, get going.

12

12. DRINK WATER / HAVE MORE LIQUID

For a long time I was suffering with a condition due to lack of drinking water. I never felt thirsty because I was seldom outdoors and hence there were days when I would just drink a glass of water or two. It was not something that I did intentionally, I just never realized it. I had digestion problems, irregular bowel problems, skin problems but I never suspected that it was all because of my lack of drinking water.

Water is a miracle fluid. You do not gain weight by drinking it but it provides you with numerous health benefits. When I finally realized how much important water is for the body, I made a conscious effort to drink plenty of water. You would never find me without a water bottle at work. I carry it wherever I go so I am not left thirsty.

Lot of people in the US drink ice cold water and there is lot of debate regarding the benefits of warm water vs. ice cold water. I wouldn't go into the details of that because none of the studies have proved either of them as bad. I personally drink lukewarm water and lots of them just because drinking lukewarm water cools the body. I also lost five pounds without doing anything other than drinking plenty of lukewarm water in just a few months.

My body's metabolism which was idle for quite some time started working up and I believe the increase in metabolism due to the consumption of water was the reason for the additional five pounds that I lost. Water is one thing that you can take without worrying about side effects. It will provide you numerous benefits like regulating your body temperature, aiding in digestion, increasing your metabolism but not a single bad effect.

In addition to water, I would like to spend some time stressing the importance of fluids. As a rule of thumb always remember that taking liquids always is easier for body to digest than solids excluding alcohol of course. So it is a good idea to start incorporating lots of fluids in your diet like soups, freshly squeezed juices, smoothies, teas and so on. Starting your meal with a bowl of soup helps in curbing your hunger, gives you a feeling of being full and hence you do not end up eating lot of food. Having a bowl of soup with some protein is ideal but I will leave it up to you to play with it. It is always a good idea to reach for liquids rather than solids when in need of a snack.

13

13. TREAT YOURSELF

Losing weight is not all about giving up. It is also about getting rewards. Other than the obvious reward of a great and healthy body which is a long term treat, you also need to periodically reward yourself with some short term treats. We all love sugar, fats and unhealthy food. That is the reason all that food industry is surviving and in fact doing pretty good.

Three chapters back when I asked you to create your own regimen, there is one point that I missed deliberately. That was the part about rewarding yourself. As part of your regimen you should also allocate sometime to relish the foods (unhealthy foods) that you love. I never use the word hate ever in my writing. It gives a very negative feeling. And so no matter how unhealthy and bad a particular food is, if you love it you should reward yourself with it occasionally with your favorite dessert or Frappuccino or hamburger.

There is however a fine line between rewarding and making it a habit. For example an occasional hamburger won't harm you but if you start having it twice or thrice a week that too in the evening, then you are doomed to go down.

The easiest way to manage this is to keep a personal milestone. For example set a target to achieve in terms of your weight loss goal and when you get to that goal, reward yourself with an additional margarita or hamburger or whatever it is that you like. That doesn't mean that you take four to six months to achieve your target. Most people cannot wait that long and give into the temptation. Set a target that you can achieve within four to six weeks instead. It doesn't have to be losing five pounds. It can be something as simple as achieving five hours of physical activity in a week.

Many people fail and give up because they set the wrong targets. No matter what you do in life, do it in increments. Set small targets, achieve it and move ahead. It gives you a sense of accomplishment, you get to retrospect on what went wrong and what went right and it also encourages you to move forward rather than giving up. Follow this not just for your weight loss but for anything else that you wish to undertake in your life.

14

14. WHAT ABOUT WINTER?

Winters are probably our worst enemies when it comes to losing weight. The weather is cold, sometimes even snow and rains, daylight is short which means lesser time to go out and on top of all that we have the big holiday season which involves a lot of heavy eating. From Halloween to Thanksgiving to Christmas and New Year, and if you are lucky, you get to celebrate a few other festivals too like Eid, Diwali, Hanukkah etc.

At the end of all this we are left with our stomach full and a few extra pounds by the end of December. Well let me tell you some interesting facts about winter. Contrary to most people's belief, winter is a time when you can lose weight easily both scientifically and otherwise too. Surprised? Let me elaborate more.

Needless to say everything goes dormant in winter, so does our body too. But that's not bad news. Apparently, our body burns more calories in winter trying to digest the food that we take and keep us warm. But that doesn't mean you can eat anything and everything to your hearts content. Winter does make one more hungry and there is this constant urge to eat more. The best way to deal with it is to drink lots of fluids, tea (with no sugar of course), soups, warm water etc.

Now let's talk about maintaining our daily regimen, remember working out at least thirty minutes per day that we promised earlier. How do we go about maintaining that? The sun sets before 5pm which means it gets dark by the time you get home. And if you live in a place where it snows a lot then that's the end of it.

Well the easiest way to overcome that is by exercising at home. As much as I enjoy going out for walks and running in the park during spring and summer, I do tend to skip doing it every day because I often make other plans like meeting up friends, catching movies, hitting the mall and so on. But in winter I rarely make plans to go out. I like to sit at home with heater on. But what to do with all the time left in my hands. Well, I use it for my 30minute regimen. I do make it a point to work out at home every day for 30 minutes.

There are many ways to work out at home, for example climbing stairs, walking around the house, dancing etc. Pick any one or even all of them but make sure to do it every day. I usually play reruns of my favorite TV sitcom and walk/jog around the house as I watch/listen to it. It's a fun way to time my exercise and also not get bored of walking around the house again and again in circles.

Eat to your hearts content during winter but make sure to follow the 30 minute rule every day, if possible change it to 45 minute rule during winter to compensate for those extra cookies that you will gobbling during holiday season.

15

15. BINGE EATING

How many of you can claim that you do not binge eat? I am guessing not many of us can answer that positively. Most of the time we are in situations when there are lots of food, good food, favorite food and leftover food. All this is accompanied by the fact that there is an occasion to celebrate and there are plenty of people around us to encourage us to eat more and more. What happens next is known to all of us. We eat not just to our hearts content but even more.

Special occasions, parties, weddings, holidays such as Thanksgiving and Christmas provide us with lot of temptations. There are plenty of food most of which are either loaded up with sugar or fats (bad fats). We prepare all year round just so that we can eat on these occasions. Most of us give into the temptation hoping to make up for it later by working out a little more. But who are we kidding here, that never happens unless you are really conscious, in which case you wouldn't be reading this book.

Anyway, there are few rules that I follow to curb binge eating (I never binge eat at any time):

1. Always leave the table when your stomach is half full: I do this because even after lunch or dinner is over, people will often offer you dessert, beverages which you need room for.

2. If there is leftover either freeze it and eat it after a week or two or pack and give it away. Lot of people give the excuse of having tons of leftover food and do not want to waste it so they end up gobbling as much as they can to avoid the food from getting waste.

Well, first of all your stomach is not a garbage bag and second you are not doing anyone favor by finishing off the leftover food. Yes, kids in Somalia are dying of hunger but you eating the leftover food will not help them in anyway. Stay healthy and do something real for the kids rather than feeling guilty.

3. Learn to say no: Yes, it's your mom and she will feel good if you eat that extra pie but it doesn't hurt to say no. I have been in such situation like a million times. Do not give in to the emotional threatening of mom's or anyone else, instead tell them you will have it couple hours later or even better ask them to pack some for you so you can relish it tomorrow when you aren't so full.

4. Cook only enough for you to eat: Most of the time the reason we eat more is because we cook more or order more food. Always cook lesser than what you always eat or twice the amount and use it for two meals. Most people who live alone face this problem as they find it hard to cook for one person.

16

16. PEER PRESSURE

Peer pressure can play a huge role on your eating habits. After all who we live with and spend time with everyday has a considerable impact on what we become and that includes our body weight. Yes, you read it right; food habits are greatly influenced by the place we live and the people we hang out with.

I remember when I first moved to the US, I was shocked that waiters don't serve water in restaurants unless you ask for it. I also noticed that almost everyone I went out with during my first few days used to order coke or lemonade to drink instead of water. In fact I did not even know that asking for water was a valid option. Within two weeks, I felt like my body has more coke than water. That is when I realized that I needed to stop drinking soda (aerated beverages) before it gets out of hand.

Well that was one of the first things I stopped after coming to US. I stopped drinking soda; instead I get water (no ice) with lemon on it. This is something that I am very proud of and often use it as an example to inspire my friends who are trying to quit soda. Most of them like me were occasional soda drinkers but after joining work and going out with colleagues for lunch every day, they got addicted too.

Another example of peers influencing your food is eating junk. For about a year, I went out for lunch with my colleagues. And in an attempt to add variety, my colleagues ended up trying different restaurants and putting lots of junk food into their stomach. Like for example Subway sandwich on Day 1, Burrito on Day 2, Hamburger on Day 3, Mediterranean Kabobs on Day 4, and Vietnamese Pho on Day 5 and so on. I went along with this routine for a while until I realized this was not doing any good for me both financially and health wise. Instead I went home made my own sandwich with whole wheat bread custom made with the right portions of veggies, meat, almost no cheese or dressing or may be a dash of the dressing and a bowl of fruits. I mentioned earlier about adding variety to the diet but trying out five different cuisines in the same week is not the way of adding variety.

Another example of peer pressure is office lunches. I used to work for this project where they provided free lunch and dinner. Lunch at 11.30 am, sometimes as early as 11.15 and dinner at 5.30pm. I typically used to have my breakfast at 9am, lunch at 12.30 and dinner by 7 or 7.30pm. But with this project on my hand my schedule was out of whack. Plus every meal was a new cuisine so instead of five cuisines a week, it was ten cuisine a week in this case.

I soon realized this was no good. So as soon as lunch was served, I used to head out for a short break at noon and went straight home for my homemade food. This way I got the break that I needed and avoided eating unhealthy food. That doesn't mean I did not eat at work at all. Certain days when the food was really good and something that I wanted to try, I would have it there. One important thing to consider here is that there were some people in the project who ate at home and ate the food at work also just because they like it. Avoid doing this at all costs. Never binge eat.

Here is another example. I had a roommate few years ago who add odd eating routine. She once got hungry at 4pm. I had just finished my lunch around 2pm and wasn't hungry but just because she was my friend and wanted me to accompany her out, I went along and had to gobble some French fries as she feasted on some wings and fries. I did this for quite some time until I bumped into another common friend. Around six to eight of us had gone clubbing that night and on our way back all of us were hungry, we decided to stop by at Denny's Restaurant and each of us ordered something to eat and drink except for this friend who said she will just have water. When I asked her why she isn't eating, she mentioned she doesn't eat that late in the night and would go home and have cereal instead. That was a moment of enlightenment for me. I did not know that was even an option. From then on, I stopped ordering food just because others I accompanied were hungry.

Don't do things just because others are doing it and this is important not just for your diet and health but in anything you do in your life.

17

17. It takes time

This chapter serves as an ice breaker to other chapters. Until now you have learnt a lot and probably even got bored by reading about what to eat, what not to eat, how much to eat, when to say no, how to identify good food vs. bad food, exercise, sleep and so on. In this chapter I will not focus on any techniques. In this chapter I will tell you a story.

This is a story about a person who was very impatient. He always thought that he is never successful. He worked very hard but no matter how much he worked, he faced failures again and again. Just when he thought he was about to achieve something good that would make his life, something bad would happen and he will have to start life all over again.

This is also taken from my first book 25 Short Stories for all ages.

> *Once there was a man who was a firm believer of God. He was brought up in an orthodox family and had learned that everything in life happens*

for good, though he himself wasn't very lucky. He was a very sincere person but for some reason things did not work out very well for him.

Right from his childhood he used to be the nicest kid but when it comes to getting caught with a mischief or owning up to a prank; he would be the one paying for it. He would never complain when things won't work the way he wanted as he always thought that there would be something better waiting for him later.

Things continued the same way as he grew up. He was doing well in high school and suddenly he had a terminal illness due to which he missed out on a lot of classes which affected his grades and he was denied scholarship in a college that he wanted to go.

He ended up going to community college and just when he was about to take up a good job in the city, his father died and he had to stay back at home to take over his father's business and take care of his mother. He left his dream job and took charge of his father's farm although he never liked working in the farm.

After few years when his business was running into heavy losses, he got a contract for a huge shipment. Although he did not have enough money to buy the raw material for the order, he took a few loans to meet the order as he thought that this order might help him make some profits in his business.

He borrowed a lot of money and bought high quality seeds and fertilizers and equipment for this order and made everything ready. But unfortunately that year his city was hit by a severe drought. He did not have water and all his saplings dried out even before they could grow.

He was devastated and completely lost faith in God. Until that day he believed that everything in life happens for a purpose but after that day he lost hope. As he was sitting at his home wondering how to pay back his loans, a person knocked on his door. He said he was interested in buying his farm.

The man sold the farm and paid all the loans and went to the city. After going to the city he contacted few of his friends and acquaintances from college and got the job that was offered before. He soon became successful in his new job and got promotions too. He earned back all the money he had lost and also got a house for himself.

It was then that he realized that he was wrong when he thought that God is not by his side. He understood the purpose for his failures. Had he not failed in his farming business and lost everything, he would not have gone to the city and taken up his dream job.

The moral of the story is to never lose hope. Being patient is a virtue and probably one of the hardest things to practice. It is nice to have dreams. Dreams give us a hope to live but one must remember that dreams don't get fulfilled overnight. Nothing happens overnight. Everything takes time and so does your goal to lose weight. Do not get disheartened if you do not succeed at first. Learn from your mistakes and come back with a better plan to achieve your goal.

18

18. WHAT TO DO WITH CRAVINGS -
FIGHTING THE MIDNIGHT HUNGER

Alright, so you followed everything this far and also got most of it right. Now what? What do you when you really crave for food or if you wake up in the middle of the night hungry? How do you stop yourself from grabbing that snack? How do you stop the temptations?

Cravings and hunger pangs are common. Most of us have to deal with midnight hunger or hunger between meals and if this is not dealt with properly then it could be a deal breaker. All your hard work, diet and regimen can go waste if you do not pay attention to this one.

Every problem has a solution and so does this one. Let's start with the root cause first. The reason you are getting hungry or having hunger pangs is a sign that you are starving or not eating well, unless you are going through some hormonal changes in which case it is normal. Other than that if you are feeling hungry between meals then it is a clear indication that you are not eating adequate amount of food in your meals. Now I know that I mentioned about portion control and eating till you feel half full but my intention was never to starve you.

One easy way to curb hunger is to eat more protein in your meals. Protein is obviously good for health but it also helps you feel full and hence you do not feel hungry for a long time. But remember too much protein is also not good for health. You need to accompany it with proper physical activity, in fact lots of physical activity. Let's say you followed all this, yet you find yourself feeling hungry. Now that your metabolism has increased you have started digesting food faster than before. What do we do now?

First and foremost if the body is hungry feed it and feed it with good food. No junk food, no fast food, feed it with proper food otherwise you will feel hungry after couple of hours again. Grabbing a quick bite from the 24x7 fast food restaurant seems like the most convenient choice at these times but never go for it at any cost. Make a quick healthy sandwich and eat or grab a fruit, whichever works best for you. The idea is to eat healthy when you are hungry.

However midnight hunger is different. The best way to curb midnight hunger is to get a sound sleep. If you are not awake then you will not be hungry. If you have your dinner at 6pm and you haven't gone to bed until midnight then you are sure to feel hungry at 12. And eating something at midnight and going to bed immediately is not good either. Best way to curb midnight hunger is to eat your dinner three to four hours before you sleep. That way you have plenty of time between your dinner and sleep and you won't feel hungry too.

Now let's talk about cravings. I usually like to eat healthy like plenty of vegetables, fruits, fish, and wheat bread and so on. But once in a while, I crave for junk food like French fries, hamburger, Frappuccino. The best way to deal with cravings is to give in to it the first time. Because the more you avoid, the more it will come to your mind and it will reach a point when all you can think of is your hamburger.

If you give in to your craving on the first day and if you still crave for it couple days later, you can at least remind yourself that you just had it the day before and motivate yourself to wait another two weeks before you can have another one. Another way to curb cravings is by using the strategy we read about in the chapter "Treat Yourself".

19

19. A LITTLE BIT OF DANCING EVERYDAY

Do you dance? If you are someone who has learnt the art of dancing and dances for a profession or for pleasure, then you may already know the magical power of dancing. But if you are like me who has never really danced in public then you may be someone who is underestimating the power of dancing. Dancing is the best thing you can do to yourself. It serves multiple purposes like providing physical activity that is much needed for your body, burning calories, relieves stress which in turn improves your mood and of course makes you a good dancer.

If you are still thinking about how to include that 30 minutes of physical activity in your regimen every day without including those boring long walks or running on the treadmill then this could be the thing for you. The beauty of dancing is that it can be done anywhere anytime like in your garage, in your bedroom, living room, kitchen, gym, and park or even in the subway. You do not need equipment, usually your iPod or headphones is enough and you can start doing it anywhere anytime.

Although it is good to learn a particular style of dance, but let's not change focus here. What I am referring to here is an activity that will motivate you. You do not have to take dancing lessons or pay for dancing instructor unless you are preparing for dancing with the stars. If your end goal is to burn calories and also learn some dance moves then all you need is YouTube. There are plenty of dance videos online, specifically look for Zumba lessons or other forms of fast dancing technique and dance your way out as much as possible.

You do not have to get the step right. Remember your goal is to burn calories and have a good time not win a reality show. I usually use this technique in winter months when I am lazy to go out for my evening walks. This doesn't mean slow forms of dancing are not good. Some of the best forms of dancing like classical Indian dances are one of the best forms of meditation. It teaches you to focus and be disciplined.

Dance in any form is good. The point here is to pick up what best suits you and keep doing it. May be few weeks down the line you may really start liking it and pursue dancing on a long term basis.

20

20. CUT DOWN MEAT AND ADD MORE VEGGIE

I know people who eat meat cannot stop eating it because it's so delicious. Up until I was twenty-five years old, I was only a chicken eater and would only eat other meat occasionally. But as I grew up, I travelled different places, was exposed to different cuisines and I started trying other meat and started liking them eventually.

Meat provides proteins but at the same time fat too, especially when it's red meat. There is a reason turkey is called lean meat, because it doesn't contain fat. If you can cut down on meat, that's the best thing you can do to your body. However, I know it can be hard to give up meat so here is what I do.

I eat meat only during weekends. Rest of the days, I eat vegetables and fish. I eat egg for breakfast everyday as well as fruits. Even if you don't reduce meat, if you can start including salad with every meal and fruit for dessert, it will make a huge difference in the quality of your physical life. A tip for those who don't like vegetables, mix egg while cooking your veggies and make it flavorful.

Nutrition for body provides nutrition for the mind. Instead of ingesting dead animals how about providing something in its natural form to the body. If you cut back on the amount of red meat that you eat, it will be great. Red meat is really hard to digest and since your digestive system is one of the most energy-consuming processes of your entire body, valuable energy reserves are needlessly depleted by this foodstuff. Some of the strongest animals like gorilla and elephants do not eat meat.

Energy is precious. You do not want to waste it on burning dead meat in your body. Start by eliminating small portions of meat in your diet and slowly increase it. You will definitely notice the difference in your energy levels. I know it is hard but isn't life about overcoming temptations and self-control. If you can master the art of self-control then anything can be achieved.

21

21. HAVE A NICE BREAKFAST EVERYDAY

Nothing cheers me up better than a nice breakfast in the morning. Eggs, hash browns, sausage links, French toast, coffee anything. I don't pay much attention to what I eat for the rest of the day but I definitely make sure to start my day with a nice breakfast.

No matter how late I wake up, I will make myself a nice yummy (non-cereal) breakfast to start my day. I do like cereal but I feel it's just isn't enough to provide me with the nutrients I need to get my day started. Plus there is no variety, its plain boring. I remember the days when I was living with my parents, my mom would have the breakfast ready for me even before I woke up. Oh, how I wish she was around.

Lot of people out there skip their breakfast or do not pay enough attention to what they have for breakfast. When it comes to breakfast, there is just one simple rule - "Never skip your breakfast!!! Period". Even if the world is ending, do not forget to take a nice balanced breakfast. You can skip food rest of the day, I don't care.

A healthy breakfast helps in getting your metabolism started. Your body is starving after not having anything for the last eight to ten hours, so you better be feeding it with something good as opposed to donuts or some other sweet treats.

For those who are looking to lose weight, here is a tip. Having a nice breakfast loaded with protein and carbs will make you feel full which in turn will make you eat less during lunch. Always eat heavy stuff during breakfast since your metabolism is high in the morning and can be easily burnt by your body. Eat light and lesser portions of the rest of your meals.

Here's to a nice Breakfast!!!

22

22. How to Continue Staying Fit

The idea of this book is much beyond the techniques of losing weight. Through these small techniques that I have described in the twenty plus chapters above, I wanted to pass a very important message to all of you. I wanted to learn disciple and self-control. If you are able to achieve these two then not just losing weight, you will be able to achieve any other goal that you have been having in your mind.

Achieving the ideal weight may be easy but maintaining it is most difficult. Here are some of the key areas that you may want to focus at:

Cook at home: One of the best ways to eat healthy is to cook your own food and eat. You can reduce the amount of salt and sugar. You can add the healthy ingredients and most important portion control. Cooking also acts as a stress reliever activity and gives a sense of satisfaction to eat nice home cooked meal.

Read the label: Never buy foodstuffs without reading the label. Always check the label, pay special attention to the amount of sodium and sugar on it.

Don't give in to temptations: Temptations will keep following you wherever you go and every time you try to do something different. These don't stop. You will have to take charge, don't let your mind drive you, you should drive the mind.

Find healthy options: Find healthy options to things that you like. May be the traditional way of eating vegetables and fruits doesn't taste good to you but there are many cuisines that make really good and appealing vegan and vegetarian dishes.

There is a restaurant chain in California named Veggie Grill. They serve fake meat, basically hamburger without the ham but soy and other healthy substitute. They also have fake varieties of chicken wings, chili and so on. Once I took my brother to this restaurant and made him try the chicken plate and wings without letting him know that it was fake meat. At the end of the day while returning back home I told him that all he ate this evening was vegan. He was startled and his expression was priceless.

The point is, it's all in your mind. If you can make your mind feel satisfied then you won't crave for unhealthy foods.

Reward periodically: Always remember losing weight is never about diet and giving up. If you like something you should have it. Come up with a reward schedule, set achievable short goals and reward periodically. Do not keep yourself away from things that you like. This is not about making you hate food or hate your life, this is about helping you control and make the right judgment of when to eat what.

Experiment: Last but not the least, keep changing your regimen. There is no one step recipe for success. It keeps changing with time. Keep experimenting with it otherwise you will get bored and stop doing it. Make it a fun experience and you will experience lifelong pleasure.

OTHER HELPFUL TIPS

If you have read my other books then you might know what this section is for. This last section is for ideas that did not make it to the main chapters as well as to get user feedback. So basically if there are ideas that you have in mind which you think needs to be included in the book, then feel free to email it to me and I will include it in a new version.

Here are some of the ideas that I feel are helpful. Some of them are not limited to weight loss but help you grow as a person.

1. **Make your bed after waking up**

    How many of you make your bed after waking up in the morning? Do you leave the bed as a crumpled mess until you arrive back home in the evening and go to sleep again in the mess? Sometimes, something as simple as making your bed in the morning after you get up can teach you to be disciplined. It can go a long way to teach us how to continue to do things. Weight loss is all about discipline. If you can control yourself from eating the unhealthy foods and convince yourself to do the 30 minute physical activity no matter what, you will go a long way in your effort to lose weight.

2.   Find a friend

Some people believe that following the weight loss regimen along with a friend encourages them to be on top of it and do it even better. You can plan on the physical activity together and also act as a police to each other by stopping them from falling into temptations.

3.   Join a club

Sometimes joining a club which encourages people to hike every weekend or bike to the mountains or participate in a marathon or something as simple as walking in the trail nearby can give you the inspiration to do the work. There are some people who don't like to do things alone and no matter how many friends you have, there can be situations when you do not find anyone to help you with your regimen. This could be a solution to your problem.

4. Invest in a good running shoes

This is one investment that you will never regret. Doing long hours of physical activity with improper gear can harm you more than providing you with any benefit to your body. The last thing you want is end up with a bunch of sores on your body. Invest on sports clothing and shoes. This also encourages you to use them and go out there rather than having them lie in your closet and accumulate dust.

5. Create more awareness

Talk about eating healthy and living healthy to your friends and family and colleagues at work. Spreading the awareness is your small way of thanking me as well as giving back to the community. Moreover when you talk about it, you may also end up finding better ways to stay healthy. Always spread the message.

EPILOGUE

I hope with the above techniques, you were able to gain some awareness about losing weight in the right way. My idea of coming up with this book is to spread the awareness. You do not have to start following them right away. If after reading this book, all you do is assess your eating habits and lifestyle, it will be a great step forward.

Progress begins in small steps. You do not have to do everything together. You do not have to be harsh on yourself. Remember no matter how you chose to do it, make it a pleasure activity. If you don't love it, you will never be able to do it.

Sacrifices are important at every stage of life. They remind us of our goals and at the end give us a sense of accomplishment. So during the course of this activity if you had to sacrifice something that you really liked then think of it as a gift you gave to yourself for your betterment.

Only great people have the courage to sacrifice, you could be one of them.

Lastly, I would like to wish you all good luck with your goals and always remember to focus on eating right not eating less.

OTHER BOOKS FROM THE AUTHOR:

25 Short Stories For All Ages

This book consists of stories which would provide an inspiration to people of all ages. Be it a young kid or an adolescent child, a college student or a young working professional, a family man or a man fighting illness. Some of the stories are inspired by real life events while some are my imagination. There is a story for everyone to feel connected to.

Small Things in Life That Can Make You Happy

When I look around, I see lot of grief and sadness. I see lot of great, wonderful, talented people - who if provided the right guidance can be one of the most happiest and successful people in this place. This book provides all such people an insight on being happy. It teaches them how easy it is to be happy. This book is a compilation of various techniques that worked for me in becoming a happier person and for those around me whom I have observed transforming into a happier and better human being.

WHAT OTHERS SAY:

Quite an accomplishment for a first time author. This
book is a good start for the author's writing career.
Stories are of the right size - neither too long nor very
short. This helped in keeping the book away after
completing a story, to get other things done and return
to read the rest.
Some of the stories are literally open-ended, leaving the
conclusion to the imagination of the reader.

-     By Amazon Reviewer

Great story. Brought a smile to my face!

-     By Blogger

Thanks for helping out, excellent information.

-     By Blogger

FOLLOW THE AUTHOR'S BLOG

CASTLEDALE.WORDPRESS.COM

CONTACT THE AUTHOR AT:

castledale.blogs@gmail.com